THE EASY WAY
TO BECOME
SKINNY FOR LIFE!

Change your mindset
and have success now

By Camilla Kristiansen

Copyrights © 2016 by Camilla Kristiansen

http://camillakristiansen.com

TABLE OF CONTENTS

CHAPTER 1: WHY YOU NEED TO BE SKINNY!

Why do you need to be skinny? You don't. That is the thing really. You don't need to be skinny, you need to be healthy, to have a body you like and love and that supports you in your everyday life. But with being skinny comes many good things. You will feel lighter, stronger, more alive and have energy to chase your kids or run after you dog or just have enough breath to walk up the stairs to your apartment. Some may argue with mer here and say that you can have all those thing without being skinny, yes for sure. I can't. I choose to be skinny. I choose to not numb myself with unhealthy food all the time. I eat what I want to and then stop.

That is the thing, you can be skinny if you want to. If you don't want to, then this book is not for you. That is ok. Stop reading right now. The only thing I want with this book is for you to figure out why you eat, and rather go out and have success in all areas of your life. Because you can. I am an entrepreneur, coach, mentor, author, stylist. I do what I feel called to the most and I know that when I'm depressed or not in alignment, I eat. Tons. Chocolate, potato chips, tons of crap and I eat to stop myself from going all in with what I want. I eat also to get over my feelings on what I really want. This is the big thing to ask yourself. Why do you have a need to be skinny? Your life will not be better when you're thin.

You will have the same problems and you will not be more capable to do more things in your everyday life, you have to admit that you wanting to be skinny is something more. Why do you have a need for it? What lies underneath? For me it's about feeling healthy, feeling toned and sexy. I want to run easily after my kids, be strong and lift heavy stuff, I want to easily get into my size S in all my clothing. So I decide on it. That is the only thing you can do right now. Decide that you will be skinny and then it will happen. It is also all about your mindset. Feel skinny now, today and ask what would a skinny person do now? Eat? Act like? Feel like? What choice would she have on a everyday basis and what would she do when she is offered tons of unhealthy food?

Non of us are stupid. We understand now what food is good for us and what's not. We are not morons. We know what to eat, but sometimes we choose to eat unhealthy all the time. On the weekends I eat more unhealthy, but then when Monday comes I go back to my eating habits again.

Yoghurt in the mornings, bread and fruit for lunch and dinner as usual. I don't think about what to eat, I think about that I'm looking forward to eat. I am hungry when my next meal comes. That can also be a thing, that you never get hungry because of all the snacks you have in between. Do you need it? No. Or ask all the magazines that gives you advice on what to eat, then you definitive need snacks. I have decided that I don't snack that much. I like to wait until my next meal. That's it. I want to be skinny because I like to fit into my clothing, feel lighter, brighter and always fit into size S. Is it a vanity thing? I guess so, but I have decided that this is how it will be for me, and then it will be so.

What do you decide on? How much weight would you be happy with? Why is it important for you to be skinny? The thing is that you can trick your brain to think thin, be thin and always choose the right thing. It is a habit like with everything else. Having a amazing body, starting your own business, find the love of your life. Everything will be the way you tell it to. You decide in your mind and then think the way you want to. I was much heavier before I got my kids. After I had my first daughter everyone told me that I could not get back in shape again. Fuck them I said to myself. I started to work out again, eat more healthier and then suddenly all my weight was gone. Then I had another daughter and put on almost 20 kg and lost that weight also.

It took me a long time to understand that I could decide on the weight I wanted to have, eat the things that I felt called to and work out for only 20 min 3 times a week. My plan in life is to make it easy. Everything has to be easy for me. Being skinny is easy when you choose so.

Ask yourself why you're not skinny now. Is it really because you stuff your face with food? Can it be so that you are eating instead of going after what you want in life? I ask because I have done it myself. For so many years I stuffed my face with food because I felt sorry for myself, I was not aligned with myself, with my core true message in life. I went to that 9-5 job, got back home, did the same old boring stuff and then it was time to follow my dream. I was so flat out tired I just wanted to eat, to feel good for only 5-10 minutes until the bad reaction came along. I knew that it was wrong, but I could not stop it.

It was so good to just feel sorry for myself for a moment and then I watched some tv-shows and the day was over. The next day went by as usual. Same thing over and over. And then I went on a diet. Eat very well, work out 5 times a week until 2 weeks in and then I cracked. I have done it all. It can't be done with going on that diet. You have to change your life, then you will be skinny. Then you have no need to eat the whole chocolate box. Then you can take 1 or 2 and be happy with that. Now when I'm writing this I'm in Oslo airport on my way to London. I have eaten a baguette and had a bottle of water, then I will have a fruit on the plane and dinner when I'm at my arrival.

I love to travel and I can eat healthy stuff like nuts and protein bars if I feel hungry. Everything in moderation is my motto now. It is easy if you only choose to be skinny, choose to be healthy and fuel your body with vitamins and healthy stuff. I love vegetables, I love fruit, but I also love chocolate and good stuff. I can eat 1 or 2 bites and then I'm satisfied. Now I am happy about my life, I feel alive, I do what I love on an everyday basis and then I'm happy. I don't need to numb myself with food anymore. I choose the right food, but indulge when I feel called to.

I choose to be skinny because I can, so can you. Choose it because you want to, don't let anyone else force you to do anything you don't want to. This is your life, you can do whatever with it, same goes with your body. Take care of your body and your health. You only got one.

Take that kind of success you have in any area of your life and put that into eating healthy and choosing to be skinny. I know for sure I go all in with everything that means something to me. My health, my kids, family, husband, business, writing, body, health, friends. I do what it takes to ask myself every single day "how do you want to feel today?". Then I act accordingly. I take time to work out 3 times a week for only 20 minutes. Then I take a walk out in nature when I feel called to. I choose to eat healthy on an everyday basis and indulge when I want to. That's it.

Why do you need to be skinny? Ask yourself why it is important for you and choose accordingly everyday your life, your health and your happiness. You can do this. You are worth it. It is your body you choose how to let it work for you. It is not about you being vain, it is about you having a happy life where you can have it all.

Go for it now.

CHAPTER 2: WHY DO YOU EAT?

So that is the question. Can you honestly tell me why you eat? I know it is a pretty silly questions, but it is needed because most of us don't eat because we are hungry. Right? Most of the time we eat to cope with stress, fears, feel sorry for ourselves. We eat just to numb ourselves. I know, I have totally been there and I can honestly say that I can fall back again pretty quickly if I'm in a bad mood. If I feel that the whole world is against me I just want to escape with candy, chocolate and get under the duvet and feel sorry for myself.

The problem with doing that is not that big of a deal, if you only do it once in a while. The problem is when you do this every single day and rather eat than deal with your problem, then it will become an issue for you.

We all want to live a long healthy life and have some fun while we do it. Let's say that you want to try this eating thing and only eat when you're hungry. How can you start to cut back then? Well, first you have to ask yourself and really get to the bottom of your problems. Why do you eat? Answer that. Do you really need a full bag of potato chips? I don't think so.

Sometimes we eat in front of the tv and don't know how much we have eaten until it is too late. So be conscious when you eat. I use to only put how much I plan to eat on a plate and then stick to that. Then you will not over eat. If you feel the urge to go back and grab more, then ask yourself why you need it? Why can't you be satisfied with the portion you just eaten up?

Then go to the core of your problem. Your feelings is messing with you. Your body don't need snacks. Your brain needs it. Why? Ask until you get there to the core. Rather than dealing with issues around feeling unhappy, you eat. Rather than going after your dreams, you eat. Rather than going to the gym, you eat. Rather than quit your boring 9-5 job, you feel sorry for yourself and eat. Rather than dealing with difficult people in your life, you eat. Rather than taking full responsibility of your life, your health, you blame it on others and eat.

I know it all. I have done it all. I have eaten when I lost my babies when I was pregnant, I have eaten when I felt trapped in my 9-5 job, I have eaten tons of candy when I should dealt with myself and just gone after my dreams.

I can't tell how many times I have picked up a bag of potato chips and eaten the whole bag and numbed myself for a few minutes. Then the guilt comes and you feel sick and even sorrier for yourself. The problem is not you, the food. The problem is that you would rather blame it on someone else and NOT deal with the real issues that are going on inside of you. Maybe you eat to have control, maybe you eat to get over horrible things that has happened to you, maybe you eat to escape your life. Instead of eating crap you could choose to nourish your body with healthy food and take a walk outside in nature and ask yourself what do I really want with my life?

I believe that people numb themselves with food because they want to escape. Life has gotten so hard and it is difficult to change it. The thing is that you can change your life right now in this moment. As long as you are willing to look the beast in the eye and tell it to fuck off.

You don't need all that crappy food. You want to be healthy, live a life in freedom where you can call the shots and go to the gym when you feel like it, not because you are guilty of eating to much crappy food. You are supposed to indulge when you want to, but then go back to your healthy eating habits again straight after. Life is beautiful, you can do, be and have anything you want to if you only open up for it and let it in.

Take a walk out in nature and breath in the fresh air, eat because you want to give your body nice fuel and take a closer look at your life. Are you happy? If not then change it. Tell yourself that you will change it today and that you are over with the unhealthy eating habits. It is only your mind that plays tricks with you so you can stay safe and NOT go after your dreams. Magic can happen you see. Your ego want you right where you belong, in the safe spot, hiding and not going after your dreams.

For so many years I did eat tons of crappy stuff. I felt so awful and fat and did not want to go out in public. I was not fat, but I FELT fat. I did work out only because I wanted to be thin and get back in shape. I pushed myself to go to the gym even if I did not feel like it. I was bored and nothing was working out. Yes, I did get back into shape again after a while, but then in the summer all the weight got back again. It was the same thing over and over. Every summer.

My twenties was not good at all. I was lonely, felt like a fool, felt that life is something that only happen to me and that I could not control it. I started to read self-help books when I was 22 and boy did I need them.

My life changed when I saw that I was the only one that could take full responsibility for my life. I said that I wanted to start my own business, follow my dreams and make them happen. I was destined to make it. Then when I was pregnant twice and lost the babies I felt that life was unfair. I wanted to die. What was the point, nothing was working and my business never took off. I felt like a failure, a fraud and a bad woman. Could not be pregnant again and give my youngest daughter a sibling. It was a horrible time. So to cope with that, I eat. More food, more crappy candy. I numbed myself until I said to myself that I'm over it. I started to take action towards the things I wanted and just picked myself up again and again.

I did get pregnant again and after I had that baby I wanted to get back in shape again, for life. It is possible to get into shape again after you have had kids. It is possible to go after your dreams and don't numbs yourself with food and other stuff to NOT have to look at your life and take action. Life is happening right in this moment, don't let the food be the thing that takes away your life from you. You can think yourself thin. I have done this and the first step is to decide what you want and how you want it. I have decided on that I will only eat 3 meals a day, I will include fruit in my lunch and have vegetables on my dinner plate.

In the weekends I can indulge on candy and other unhealthy stuff, but then I go back to eating healthy on Monday. I will only work out 3 times a week for only 20-30 min. I want my exercises to be quick and fun. I will not do anything I feel is boring. Then I will walk out in nature everyday if I have the time, not to be slim, but to clear my mind and tap into my intuition.

That is it. I can't deal with diets and working out at the gym for hours. This is my plan and when I decided that this will work, it did. I am now much more slimmer than I was before I got the kids. The only thing I did was to decide on how I wanted it. Then I followed that plan and it worked out. Ask yourself today how you want your plan to be and stick to that. Believe that you can do it and you can. Affirm daily that "I'm now so grateful that I'm healthy, weight .... and love my life". Then so it will be.

CHAPTER 3: THE 20 MINUTE RULE

This is how you really can focus on all the things in your life you want to change. 20 min is all it takes. Too good to be true? I don't think so. Let's say you want to set aside 20 minute to everything that means something in your life right now. For me it's my health, my business, my kids, husband, relaxing time, write on my books etc. The thing is that we all got 20 minutes. Even if I have kids I don't need to sit and hold their hands all day long. I can set aside 20 minutes and clean the house. When 20 minutes is over then I'm done. The thing is if you set a time for when you will finish a task, that will be the time it takes.

I do this when I write a blog post, when I write on my books and when I work out. I set aside 20 minutes 3 times a week right after I have eaten my lunch. I find work out videos on YouTube and follow a program I love. For me it must be fun, or else I wont do it. I have tried to follow restricted trainers like Jillian Michaels, but it's too boring in the long run. I also switch up my workout programs every months so I don't get bored. The 20 minute rule can be used in ever area in your life. This is how you can write a book, workout, clean your house, spend time with your kids, do some boring admin tasks etc.

As long as you say to yourself it is only for 20 minutes, then it can be done. You can deal with anything for only 20 minutes. Right? When it comes to making dinner for my family, I do it myself. I plan out for a whole week what we will eat and then we do the weekly grocery shop and stick to that list. Making dinners also only take me 20 minutes. Let's say I want to educate myself more and read books or watch inspiring videos, then I set aside 20 minutes to do that. The only thing you need to do is to figure out what is most important for you on a daily, weekly and monthly basis. When you have done that then you break it down and work on those things that is important for you.

Let's say you want to write a book. Then you need to actually set aside time for that. Writing. 20 minutes each day is enough. People try to complicate things so much that they can't seem to start. When it comes to having success in any area of your life, you need to start. Get it? Start to eat healthy today, start to work out today. Don't wait for things to happen, life is what you make out if it and you are the driver in the seat of your car. You can become slim for life if you want to. Think how easy it will be when you have decided that you will only fit into size S or M or L.

The size that matters to you must come from your heart. Don't try to be thinner than you want to and can cope with. You have to give yourself a little slack and just indulge when you feel called to. As long as you don't do it on an everyday basis then you will be fine. The thing here to understand is that you must take full responsibility on your own life and set aside 20 minutes to work out, go for a walk, eat healthy, plan your meals, clean your house, follow your dreams. I promise you when you see that missing link, that is you not following your passion and your dream, you will want to stop eating. You will stop numbing yourself with crappy food and be so engaged in your own life that you don't need to eat to feel sorry for yourself.

The stress you feel today on your body, I believe, is linked to YOU not following your calling. Your passion and your big dream in life. Don't listen to the naysayers, they will never understand you. They will never take time out not even 20 minutes to think about how they want to improve their lives.

The negative people use tons of time to be NEGATIVE. So please don't listen to them, do this by your own and write down how you want your life to look like. Don't think about the how. The same goes for your weight. The weight or scale will figure it selves out when the WHY is strong. Understand yourself and why you want to be thin. Why is it important for you and set aside 20 minutes to work on that. Your eating habit, work out routines, take a walk out in nature, join a gym. Whatever you can do to lift your mood up and just be happy. Life is supposed to be lived with joy and happiness.

It has actually only taken me 20 minutes to write this chapter. Then I can keep going and write for 20 minutes more or I want to get something else done. I have already done my 20 minutes work-out for today. Then in the evening I have to admit that after the kids have gone to bed I want to eat. I want to reward myself with something sweet. Before I could eat a whole chocolate plate, now I can take 3 bites and be fine with that. Then I write some more on my books or take a walk out in nature or just relax and watch a series on Netflix. Let yourself have balance in your life and don't be too hard on yourself. We are only human and of course we can have anything we want in moderations.

As long as we are in balance with our feelings we will be fine.

We have to get past those things that are holding us back, those deep things that we only tell ourselves and are afraid to admit to others. Lucky me, I can tell it all in my books and get rid of it. So can you. Write it out. Scream. Get it out. What is holding you back from living a fantastic life, having freedom, go after what you want? Only you know the answer to that. As a coach and mentor I help women to get past those blocks they have and often it is things from their childhood that has been holding them back for years.

You have to understand that you are good enough. You are more than capable to say NO to candy and other crappy food. You have the power inside, and when you are ready to only focus on those areas in your life for 20 minutes each day then the magic happen. Most people THINK that it will not work. So they don't try. They are right. As long as they don't try, it will not work. That's it. You have to try, start and get over your fear of not being good enough. You are more than good enough and you can do this. Being thin is easy when you know how to think and how to act. Just focus on the good stuff in life and then you don't need food.

Food is there to nourish us, make us grow and we need it to function. We need food so don't deprive yourself from it. Eat the right one and you will never need that much crappy food in your life anymore. You will want to focus on your goals in life rather than numbing yourself with food.

Just say to yourself that "now it's time to take full charge in my life, live it to the max". Then you start for 20 minutes and focus. And then when 20 minutes are gone, you are done. If you want to work more then fine, do that. But don't force yourself and let your ego tell you that 20 minutes is not enough. It wants you to never be done, you are never good enough for your ego. It wants you to play safe and hold yourself back so no one can touch on you. But you know that your growth will happen outside of your comfort Zone.

You need pain to grow. Pressure. Uncertainty. Trust. Faith. Just do it. Start today and plan out for your success. Don't give up until you know how you want to design your life. You can plan it out as much as you want to, but if you never take action towards it, then it will never happen. You have to make it happen now. Don't wait. Plan it now. You can do this. I believe in you.

One life, live it to the max.

CHAPTER 4: INSTEAD OF NUMBING YOURSELF, DO THIS!

You know it so well that you eat only to escape. You don't need all that food. I'm sick and tired to pat you on your head. Can you see that YOU are the only one that can make it happen? You can stop numbing yourself with food. You don't need it. How much longer are you going to stick your head in the sand and say that you will be over now. You will not do that again? I don't believe you. Instead of numbing yourself with food then do this.

Think.

For.

Yourself.

Stop asking me or anyone else how it is done. What are you talking about? You know it all. Food is there to fuel you up, not to help you get over your problems. You need a pat on the head and someone that says that you will be fine, everything will be fine in the end. It will not. As long as you are not willing to take full responsibly on your life, your body, your food, it will not happen. Nothing happens by chance. You have to be willing to work for it. Your body, your health, your dreams. Everything you want is right there in front of you, but instead you want to eat. Sit there on the couch and feel sorry for yourself. Who are you kidding? Don't you think we can see you, notice you how you have been holding back.

It's only your life. Right? Only one chance to have that hot, sexy body you long for, or not. Maybe you don't want it that bad? Maybe you read this book and think that you will be thin by only reading about it? Can't you see that everything you tell yourself is true? The things you tell yourself is true, for you. Not for everyone else, for you. And what life are you living right now? Your own or someone else's? I don't think you care about your life, your dreams, your body. You don't give a fuck about yourself. Because if, only if, you did that would you then be sitting and reading my book about how to be thin?

You know it so very well. You know it all. How to eat. How to work out. You are not stupid. Right? At least I hope not. Sorry to be a little bitch now, but you need it. Time is out, over, stop bullshitting yourself that this time you will make it. It will not happen. You will never be thin because

a. you don't give a shit about it

b. you rather numb yourself than facing your fears.

That is it. All I have to say today. Get the fuck over yourself and ask, really fucking ask if you want it that bad? Do you? Then if you still keep on reading this book, then let's get to work. So what can you do instead than numb yourself with food?

The work.

That is needed.

Follow your passion.

Your dreams.

Stop telling yourself bullshit that you are happy, fine, will get used to NOT liking your life.

Get a grip and start to act on your dreams no. Today.

When dreams are unleashed you don't want to numb yourself

anymore. Get it? How? I don't know what you dreams are. Find them. Do it. Stop telling that you can't.

CHAPTER 5: SUCCESS HABITS

How you do one thing, is how you do everything. It is actually so easy to be thin for life. You just need to see that in one area (or more) in your life you are killing it. You know it so well and you do the fucking job. You go all in. The thing is that area in your life you really have success in, you can take those success habits and use them when you try to change your eating habits. One area in my life I have control over, and kick ass in, is my business. I am so organized and know what to do on an everyday basis and I also find time to grow my business and build my audience. The thing is that now it comes so natural for me I don't think about it anymore.

It was not like that in the beginning. In the beginning I followed everyone else and were not aligned with my message and why I wanted to have success in my business. Now I start my morning with success habits. Journaling, meditation, essential oils, write my blog, make a video and write on my books. The thing is when you have found your success system you can implement that in every are of your life. For me it's planning. Aligned planning that I love, like and know will get me to my final destination. When it comes to eating habits then make a plan for a week, what will you eat? Then stick to that plan and know that when you feel flat out tired and want to stuff your face again, have a fruit or something to get your mind on something else.

Everything can be done as long as you want it, can work to have it and align yourself towards it. You got to have some kind of success habit if you want to make money fast in your business and be successful. You already know what to focus on right now and then the next step is to actually do it. So on days when you just don't feel like it, what to do then? I guess you have to just suck it up and do it anyway. Just get to work even when you don't feel like it. That is how you will have success. And when shit happens in your life, get used to that and say to yourself that you are bigger than that problem. The truth is that every problem can be fixed and you will make it happen when you take full responsibility for your life.

You are allowed to have success and you will have it when you just do your work day in and day out even if you feel tired, sick, not well, not feeling like it. That is how you can create success in your life and in your business. On days when I feel flat out tired I have to just suck it up and start. Then I can't think of that small task as something I can't handle, I can't be bothered with. The clue is to look at the bigger picture and then act accordingly. That is how you can create success habits.

On days when I feel sick I just get up and start to work. I act anyway and then I take time off when I feel tired and have done my most important things for that day. If you force yourself to just do it you will get to your final destination. That is how it's done, that is how success will come your way. Your success habits must be that you show up, take action, work on your mindset and try to follow up on people that you want to work with.

Ask yourself, can you do more, be more and just go all in with your message every single day. The more you create, the more you make. Money will flow when you feel aligned with your message, with yourself and with your bigger picture.

Some days I feel like I can't bothered. When I have crashed my income goals for the month only 4 days in. why should I keep going then? Well, I could have just said to myself that I needed to relax, but then again I'm not working on my bigger picture just to make lot's of money and relax. I can't relax when there are so many more women out there that needs my help. Need me to tell them that they are allowed to just be themselves and go all in with that.

Your success habits will get you to your final goal in life and in business. That is why you have to keep on swinging and keep that swing even when things go bad, then swing harder. You got to get back in the ring and never be done until you're dead. Get it? Either you want it or you're just in it to make money. People ask my why I work so much, I ask them why they just go to work to work. I love what I do, I could do it for free. But I can't do it for free, then I can't have a business, then I can't help more people.

Can you see that your success habits you need is you taking action every single day, show up, ask for the sale, create, be you and then you will grow your business fast? In the beginning when I was first starting out I was so scared because I just did not know how to do it. How to do anything. But you can figure everything out, you just have to start. Comes with everything you actually want in your life and in your business.

Are you called for this life? Can you handle not knowing when you next money will flow into your account? Can you handle it? If not then you are not made for it. I think that entrepreneurs are born, not made. I think that they could learn some skills, but they have to have that kind of mindset that not the normal people have. They will do whatever it takes for as long it takes and some more. They will go all in and then some more. Get it? Is that you? If not the quit. Quit right now and stop telling yourself that you will make it. Because you will not. Either you're in it to win it or you are out.

You must be willing to look the beast in the eyes when you feel scared, not ready, not good enough, when people talk you down, when you can't be bothered, when you feel tired, flat out bored and just don't want to be bothered. Well, then you need to make up your mind if you really want this life? Could you keep swinging when everything feels hard and not in alignment? Of course you can. You are one of them. The ones that will make it. You have the power inside of you to act from alignment and take action regardless on how you feel. You will do whatever it takes for as long it takes because you are focused on the outcome. Your success habits will be you taking action and showing up no matter if you feel like it or not.

You are so sold on your mission in life and you really feel called to do it. You can't do anything else. You know that you will go all in for as long as it takes and you are desperate to make it. You know that you could help so many people with this message that you have inside of you so you can't just stop. Stop now? Is that even possible to think about? No. You will never give in because you have that success mindset now. You will have your success habits and they will give you everything you need. Money, fame, fortune and you will make it. Everything in your life is possible and you will make it.

No matter how long you have to wait, you can do it. But to really go all in an speed up your you know that everything is a choice. Choose to me rich, choose to me happy, choose to make it easy. Your mind can set you really fast up for success if you choose it. Most of the entrepreneurs that I talk to struggle to make money and struggle to make it. They choose to make it hard because that is what they have heard is needed. But then again hard? When you love what you do why do you call anything a job, hard, not fun? I love writing, not all the time but I know that I can inspire so many women to follow their dreams with my books.

Same goes for everything I do in my life and in my business. I have to do my daily writing, my daily videos, my daily work. I have to get it out of me. Now I'm soon running a VIP day in Oslo with a lovely client. Of course I'm a little bit afraid that she will not like it, but then again I know that I can help her. I'm sold on myself, but the fear will always creep up upon me. That is life. I have my success habit that I need to get done on a daily basis. Write, speak, make my videos, follow up. Track my money, do some kind of sale activities. How much? As much as I feel called to and then some. I just go all in with it and then some.

Can you commit to have success now? Are you willing to put in the work that is needed and can you tell yourself that you are allowed to make it? That you already are successful because you are trying? Just let yourself have it. Have it all because you deserve it. For sure.

My success habits for my business can easily be used to stay thin. I focus on why I want it, then I work towards it and then I understand that it will take me to my final destination as long as I do this day in and day out. There are quitting in business, there are no quitting in your life. Be patience and just stick to your plan. Get it?

CHAPTER 6: HOW YOU DO ONE THING IS HOW YOU DO EVERYTHING!

Think about one area in your life that you are really killing it. For me it is writing on my books, getting my content out there. I really focus on my goals in my business and I get shit done. I also am very organized when it comes to plan things out. I have a meal plan for a week and I shop only once a week. I save time and money and I am killing it in this area. Where are you a kick ass woman in your life? Is it that you are a super mum, a badass when it comes to selling, a lovely girlfriend, a loyal and nice friend? It doesn't matter what area you are good at, the thing is how you do one thing is how you do everything.

So that area in your life you are really killing in, can you apply that to your health and fitness? For sure I do it. I'm all about thing must be fun, balanced, don't take long time and mean something to me. Everything I do, I do it with ease and flow. My work outs are short but effective, I eat balanced, but treat myself when I feel called to. I take a walk out in nature to clear my mind, but I say 20 minutes is enough. So I do a lot, but the thing is that it don't take much time. Can you try to kick your own ass into action and use your success mindset in that area you are killing it, on your health and fitness?

This is how you can get skinny for life. When you know deep down that you are already that skinny person inside, you know that you only need to call her out into the open. If you can see it in your mind, you want her and you need her to step forward.

I think she has been hiding. For me it was safe and secure to have weight on my body after I had my kids. If I got skinny very fast I had to be out there and actually have success in my business. I thought I could not be a stylist if I was not thin enough and pretty enough. It was safe for me to have that extra weight on so I could just hide behind the computer and don't have success. I was so scared before to be visible, to get in front of people and speak to an audience. That was the thing with my weight. For me if I gained weight I was depressed and did not feel good. For others it might be so that they eat when they feel good.

You can apply your success mindset you have in your life to become that kick ass skinny bitch you know deep down you are. If you have a dream about it, then you can become it. You can think yourself thin if you really dig deep on how a skinny person think, sleep, act, talks, eat. It is so easy if you can start to act today as that woman. Ask yourself "what would a skinny woman as I see myself as, do on an everyday basis?". Will she force it upon herself to be thin? Will she eat unhealthy food all the time? Would she go to the gym? Will she take care of her spiritual mind also?

The thing here to really connect with her, is to write it down on a piece of paper and ask yourself how would she eat, work out, speak, talk, think, sleep, dress like, be etc. Really write everything on there that woman you see yourself as and take action on it. You have to act accordingly to this and like you are already there. If you were that woman now, how would you be then? Start to act like that. You have to really step into that mindset and become her now. Today is the first day on your new life as that skinny woman. When you feel it and act like it will come, it is the law. This is how the law of attraction can be set into actin.

Most people get it wrong when it comes to trying to loose weight. They set up a masterplan that are destined to fail. Work out every day, eat healthy all the time, push themselves to the max and try to live a life that are restricted and with boring rules. Fuck the rules. You can be thin your own way. This is the easy way. Non of us are fools. We know how to eat healthy and we know that what we put in our body must stay there or be used as energy. We can figure this out ourselves, but very often our mind trick us to be so hard on ourselves.

You can't look at your final goal as something you have to GO to. You have to see it on your mind like that you are already there. That is why how you do one thing is how you do everything will work perfect for you. That area in your life you are so good at, use those success strategies and loose weight and become skinny for life. Being skinny is healthy and easy and if you have a balanced life you will not think about food anymore. You will eat when you are hungry and when you feel bad you will deal with your feelings like it is supposed to. Not stuff your face because you feel bad.

This is your life and your body. Choose to take care of it. You have people in your life that love you just the way you are, and I suggest you love yourself right now. There is nothing wrong with you, but if you really feel that you want to be skinny, why not? You can do it. If I can do it, so can you.

I don't believe in genes and that some of us have hard time loosing weight. I believe that it is all in our mind and that we can change that if we want to.

I understand if you feel another way, that is all up to you to decide on, but I suggest you work strong on your skinny mindset and act like those skinny people do. I think that you are skinny right now, you just don't see it.

But if you feel that you want to loos 2-5 kg or more, no problem. You can do that. It is possible to think yourself thin. Get that strong mindset on right now and decide today that you will act accordingly to being that skinny woman now. You can do this. I believe in you.

CHAPTER 7: WORK OUT BECAUSE IT'S FUN!

Your body needs to move. Get off your ass and move it. Work out because it's fun. You can find something that you like to do. I only work out for 20-25 minutes 3 times a week. Those videos I find on Youtube, I change every month so I have something new to look forward too. Yes, I get bored if I do the same thing over and over again. I also love to take a brisk walk out in nature. Find something that lifts your soul and that you really like to do. You don't have to slave your ass off in a gym if you are not called to do it.

I work out because it is fun. I love it. Or I tell myself I love it?! I don't know, but you have to set your mind up for success all day long, also when it comes to getting your ass off. Just decide that you will find something that you like. Maybe it's dancing, maybe it's jogging, find something that lifts your spirit and gives you joy. Of course I don't want to work out every time, but I tell myself that everyone has 20-25 minutes to do that 3 times a week. Then I stick to that.

I have decided to do it that way and go all in with it. I can't image now that I would stop working out. I need it especially when I'm a self-employed entrepreneur that have to work in front of the computer 5-6 days a week.

I have had problems in the past with my shoulders and I also feel it now. I know how important it is to take care of yourself. Body, mind and spirit must be taken care of on a everyday basis. You can't be skinny if you never move your ass. Or you can, but it is not healthy. Your heart rhythm has to get a little bit warmed up if you want to keep your health in order. You have to understand that YOU are the number one asset in your life. You have to take care of yourself because you need it. Your family needs you to be healthy and also you need to have a healthy mindset.

Everything comes down to what you tell yourself. Do you want to work out? YES! Tell yourself you want to. Then figure out what, how many times a week and then you stick to that. Easy. In the beginning your brain wants to trick you into NOT doing it. It will tell you to stop and think that you can't do it this time. You will want to quit after a week, but if you only stick to it for 3 weeks I promise you that you are hooked. Then you can do it. Then you can stick to it for lifetime.

Of course you can change your workout routines as often as you want to. I do that.

The clue here is to understand that your body needs to move. Even if YOU (your brain) wants you to sit in the sofa, don't listen to it. You have to act like that skinny, healthy person now. Be her now. Act from that place because then you will have success fast. If you ask yourself "what would that skinny higher version of myself think now? Would she skip the work out or would she just fucking do it?" I think we both know the answer to that. So then you go all in and just act like her. Be like her. Step into that skinny persons identity now. How would she think, act, feel, speak and work out?

The fun part is that you are only a mindset shift away from becoming skinny for life. This weekend I did indulge in candy and lot's of chocolate because I have had pain in my shoulder and felt sorry for myself. Then I thought about this book, about you the lovely reader, I have to course correct myself from time to time. I'm only a human being, I do have a slip from time to time. I feel that I did eat too much candy, so I have to ask myself the next time I do this "Camilla how would you feel after you have eaten this whole bowl of candy?" Then I know how I would NOT want to feel.

So you see, we all can have a slip, but the thing is to get back to your great habits again ASAP. I do have wine and Prosecco in the weekends, but for me it's all about my mindset. The way I CHOOSE to think, be, act and feel. I have set my mind up for success the way that I have decided to work out 3 times a week. I have programmed myself to tell my body that it is enough. Your mind will keep you skinny for life if you let it have the power.

Can you do that?

CHAPTER 8: THE FRENCH WAY

I love eating the french way. Everything in moderation and with a glass of red wine. I think the french women really enjoy their food and look for quality food when they shop. They also prepare their food and make dinner for their family or go out and really enjoy eating. They eat cheese, baguette and drink red wine when they feel called to. I love the book "French women don't get fat". You should read that book and implement those thing you feel resonate with you. I feel that food should be enjoyed in moderation. That goes with everything in life. You must really enjoy life and eating. You should not feel bad because you eat a chocolate and drink red wine.

Everything in moderation, but then if it was that easy why do we eat too much? Well, that is when we are not aligned with what we really want in out lives. I remember back in college when I was not enjoying my life. I felt I was in the wrong place at the wrong time, but I could not quit. I had to finish business school because I had invested in myself and I am not a quitter. But back then when I was bored, I eat tons of food and unhealthy things. I put on a few pounds more than I was happy about. When I could not close the zipper in my jeans I was fed up. I joined the gym, started to eat more healthy and suddenly the pounds I gained was gone.

I took action but not tons of action. I did what I felt called to and really enjoyed going to the gym after a while. The french women don't like to go so much to the gym, they love to go for a walk and take the stair instead of the elevator. I love to work out now, but only 3 times a week. Then I also take an evening walk. Actually I have just been out now around the block and as I write this I have a glass of red wine. Life is supposed to be fun, and amazing. You can eat whatever you want to, but your body want nutrition food. Give it that also and the other stuff in moderation.

The french way is easy, fun and doable. Because that is it. Life must be doable, amazing and you can create it just the way you want to. This is your life, your body, take full control over it. You can say no to overeating and rather ask why do you need to eat. I know there is something else that is stopping you. You are not in alignment, you are not doing what you feel called to in life. When you love life and are energized you don't need to eat. When I have a full day of work I love, then I forget to eat. I love every moment when I write and speak and then I don't need so much food.

When you have taken full control of your life, the eating stuff will not be hard. You can think your way thin if you want to, just decide that you can eat whatever and feel that in your body. I know it sound impossible, but try it, really try it and go all in with that feeling. You design your own life and you are the driver in your own car. You can do whatever you want to and become skinny for life. It is not that hard. When you really understand that all it takes is a change of mindset, then it all will fall in place. You will not think about what to eat, you will think about going after your dreams and eat when you are hungry. You will not have a need to stuff your face with food when what you really need is to feed your soul.

My soul is calling me to write, speak and create. When I do that I can go hours without food. Same when I'm on Holiday in a warm location, I don't need that much food. I enjoy the sun, but if I get stressed I need food. Then I'm out of alignment again and need to go back to being me and my soul. It is not harder than that. It can be done and it it very easy. People complicate things a lot. French women make it easy. You can also choose to make your life easy. Give your body quality food, enjoy wine and other things in moderation and move your body daily. Feed your soul multiple times a day with soulful things you love.

Go out there and kick some ass. Your own maybe? You can do this you skinny bitch:-)

CHAPTER 9: YOUR LIFE, LIVE IT NOW!

The life you are living right now is for you to decide how you want it. The way you think about yourself, what you need to eat and not to eat is the way you will live your life. Every action you take on an everyday basis will shape the way you will look like and how you will feel on the inside. Don't you just want to take full control over your life right now because you know that you can? You don't need to eat that crappy food anymore. Find out what is triggering you to eat things to calm you down. I know when I'm stressed I need to eat to be kind to myself.

My soul needs to be heard, to be feed and then I would rather do it with my writing, my speaking and my videos than stuffing my face with unhealthy food. I know I will feel so much better tomorrow if I can just calm down a little bit and give myself what I really need. To follow my passion. When I'm out of alignment I will never ever be happy until I have eaten or worked on what my souls wants me to do. I need to be alone, have time to journal and read something inspiring. I know deep down in my heart that you will never ever be happy if you don't follow what you are called to do. I'm called to lead, speak, write, hustle, coach, show up and inspire others to go after what they want.

Sometimes I don't get it. I just don't get why people are wasting their precious times to stuff their face with crappy food when they rather could be doing what they love all day long. For me this is fuel for my soul. To write. I love it. I could do it all day long. I can do it in my sleep and I know that I could wake up 4 o clock in the morning and do it. If I really tap into my calling what I'm supposed to do, then I can do it on command. And to really know if I'm on the right path is to ask if I could do it for free? Hell yes, I can. This is my life, my future, I have created it. I have created the body I have because I see myself as thin. I have never seen myself as fat so that is how it will be. And after writing this book I guess I can never be fat again:-)

You create the lifestyle you have. You choose what to eat on an everyday basis and you have the power to just stop it. You must take control over your life and your body right now. I believe in you. Your are beautiful just the way you are right now, don't change for others. Change because you want to. You deserve it. The power you have is amazing. We all got it, but the fewest of us take advantage of it. You can decide right now in this moment that you will do whatever it takes to get into alignment so you can be skinny for life. You will not need so much crappy food then. You will be fueled on life. You will love your life.

Where in your life right now are you not stepping it up? How can you be out there more and be 100% you? Think about your family life, business, job, health, spirituality, fun time, body etc.

What can you do to really take care of yourself and do those thing that you feel are holding you back? Step it up now and take control. When you know that you are in the front seat of your life, then magic will happen. You will be so happy and thankful about your life that food will be natural for you. I know what triggers me. What triggers you?

Go all in now. You can have it all. Hot body, live your dream life and be you 100%. Just go for it.

CHAPTER 10: SKINNY FOR LIFE!

Can you really become skinny for life? Yes. Of course. You set your mind up for anything you want to se happening so if you want to be skinny, do it. I hope that this book has triggered you to think about the life you live right now. Do you live it to the fullest? Are you happy on an everyday basis? Are you doing what you are born to do? If not then what are you waiting for? When you are fully living the life you are called to do, you will not need food to calm yourself down or give yourself a little treat. Your life will be so amazing and filled with lovely moments that you will not think about eating and stuffing your face to be kind with yourself. The only thing that will really give you calmness is if you are living the life you are supposed to do.

You don't need to learn more about food. You don't need to work out more. You don't need to go on a diet. If you are truly living the life you are supposed to do then everything will fall into place. I know that when I'm stressed out it is always about me not getting what I want on an everyday basis. I need time for myself, time to journal, write, speak, create. That is all I really need. And tons of meditation, reading inspiring books and walking out in nature also gives me fuel to not stuff my face.

I have my goal for how much I want to weigh. It is actually way less than before I go the kids and was pregnant. I want you to think about your goal and go all in with it. Believe that you can be skinny, because you can. But only do it because you want to be healthy, look good and be happy in your skin. Don't do it because you don't feel good enough and pretty enough.

Decide what you want in your life and go after it. I'm not a nutrition specialist, I write about mindset and how to go after any goals in your life. Being skinny is not harder than building a business or being a good mother or a kick-ass author. You can set your mind up for success in any area of your life.

Being skinny is easy when you find out why you eat. What you eat is not that important as long as you balance it. Can you go full in now with your passion, your mind and spirit and just fucking do it? This is your life, it is happening today. Skinny or not. Here you come. Take the stage now and do it. Time will never be perfect. Start today. You can do this.

About the author

Camilla Kristiansen is a soulful mentor who helps women take action toward their big dreams and make money doing what they love. Growing up in a small town called Reine in Lofoten Camilla started her journey with a degree in Bachelor of Commerce/Business Studies and worked for 13 years in corporate jobs before she took the big leap in 2015. Later on she followed her passion in fashion and started her own business in 2010 as a stylist. Camilla now lives in Bodø, Norway with her two children and a very supportive husband. Camilla is ready to change women all around the world with her online company. Her mission is to help other women live their dream life with a business and lifestyle they love. She's all about taking action everyday to make your dreams come true. Camilla is the go to mentor for freedom seekers ready to shine!

Connect with Camilla and download her free books and videos at http://camillakristiansen.com

Get your free gift at https://camillakristiansen.com/freegift/

Learn more about Camilla at: http://camillakristiansen.com/about

Buy all of Camilla's 40+ books here: https://camillakristiansen.com/books/

Make me happy!

I will be so happy and appreciative if you'd consider leaving me feedback on this book. It will help me share my message and make other women get to know this book that can change their life in a positive way. It will only take you 2 min to leave a feedback on Amazon.

Thank you so much!

Hugs and kisses from Camilla

9 798649 524650